Beach Body Makeover: A Complete Guide to a Sexier You

Lose Weight, Get Fit and Get Healthy

Zoey Taylor

This book is dedicated to everyone struggling with weight issues, poor eating habits, negative body image issues and the lack of motivation to change it. Change your mind and you can change your body and health. You can do it - starting today!

Copyright © 2014 by Speedy Publishing LLC

All rights reserved. No part of this publication may be reproduced, distributed or transmitted in any form or by any means, including photocopying, recording, or other electronic or mechanical methods, without the prior written permission of the publisher, except in the case of brief quotations embodied in critical reviews and certain other noncommercial uses permitted by copyright law. For permission requests, write to the publisher, addressed "Attention: Permissions Coordinator," at the address below.

Speedy Publishing LLC (c) 2014
40 E. Main St., #1156
Newark, DE 19711
www.speedypublishing.co

Ordering Information:
Quantity sales; Special discounts are available on quantity purchases by corporations, associations, and others. For details, contact the "Special Sales Department" at the address above.

-- 1st edition

Manufactured in the United States of America

Table of Contents

Publisher's Notes i

Chapter 1: Tips for Getting Your Body Bikini Ready 1

Chapter 2: Finding the Right Swimwear for Your Body Type 3

Chapter 3: Ways to Increase Your Metabolism 6

Chapter 4: Fat Flushing and Increasing Your Metabolism 8

Chapter 5: Calories Must Be Burned 11

Chapter 6: Get to Know the Basics of Weight Loss 17

Chapter 7: Supplements – Are They Right for You? 23

Chapter 8: Fighting a Flabby Tummy in Search of 6 Pack Abs 25

Chapter 9: Tips on Motivation and Staying on Track 33

Meet the Author 35

Publisher's Notes

Disclaimer

This publication is intended to provide helpful and informative material. It is not intended to diagnose, treat, cure, or prevent any health problem or condition, nor is intended to replace the advice of a physician. No action should be taken solely on the contents of this book. Always consult your physician or qualified health-care professional on any matters regarding your health and before adopting any suggestions in this book or drawing inferences from it.

The author and publisher specifically disclaim all responsibility for any liability, loss or risk, personal or otherwise, which is incurred as a consequence, directly or indirectly, from the use or application of any contents of this book.

Any and all product names referenced within this book are the trademarks of their respective owners. None of these owners have sponsored, authorized, endorsed, or approved this book.

Always read all information provided by the manufacturers' product labels before using their products. The author and publisher are not responsible for claims made by manufacturers.

Print Edition 2014

Chapter 1: Tips for Getting Your Body Bikini Ready

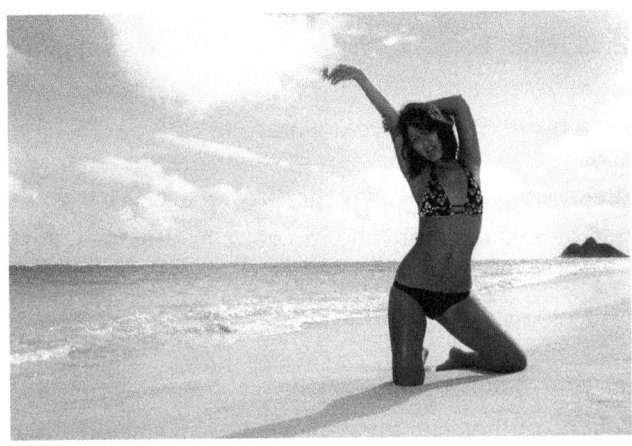

Now that summer is here, you have to take off all of those clothes that you've used to hide those less than flattering areas of your body. Unfortunately, you have a new bikini, but it looks horrible on you. But, don't worry about it because you are going to do something to get back your flattering figure.

Even if you worked out all winter, but you are still not happy with your body, then exercise to tone and firm up the flab that you've been hiding all winter long.

Conditioning exercises can do wonders to get your booty, stomach, hips and upper back toned up. You can target the areas of your body that need it the most, and tone them up by using certain exercises. Go online and look for conditioning exercise that can help you.

Now is the time to jump rope, lift weights and use the exercise ball. Using these things will get your body looking great for your new bikini. You will accomplish this by doing a little body sculpting and exercising with cardio. These things can help speed up your metabolism and burn the fat.

Drink eight glasses of water each day. This will keep you hydrated and make your skin look fantastic. You can tell if a person is eating right by looking at their skin. The water will get rid of the toxins that are in your body. It also stops the body from getting a condition known as cellulite. It is ugly and will make you look horrible in a bikini. So, drink your water.

Eat right and keep in mind that the skin reflects what you eat. So, this should be enough motivation to eat a healthy diet. Eat a lot of proteins, veggies and fruits. Also eat your carbs. This is one of the best ways to consume a healthy diet.

Now that your body is toned and looks great in your new bikini, think about all of that skin that you will be showing off. You want it to be smooth and glow all summer long. The best way to accomplish this is to exfoliate and get rid of dead skin cells. These skin cells will make your skin look tired and dry. You want soft skin that looks clean, fresh and toned. Consider using a natural bristle brush while getting rid of those dead skin cells.

Also, don't forget to remove unwanted hair from your body before putting on your new bikini. Also, remember to moisturize once it has been done. You also want to put on sunscreen while on the beach in order to combat aging and other serious conditions such as skin cancer.

If you use the aforementioned tips, you should be bikini ready in no time.

Chapter 2: Finding the Right Swimwear for Your Body Type

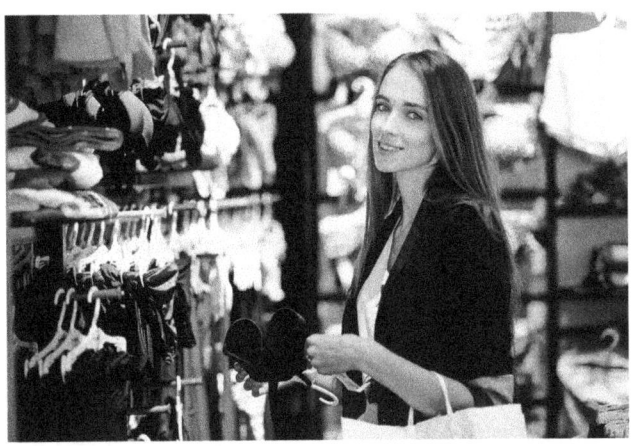

During the winter months it is easy to camouflage different parts of your body with clothes. But, during the summer months it's very hard to do. You can't keep hiding forever. It is time to admit that you have a few problematic body areas. Your winter clothes have been hiding those flabby thighs and that tire that you are carrying around your midsection. However, it'll soon be time to hit the beach for a little fun and relaxation. If you are worried about how you'll look in a swimsuit, or even worse a bikini, use the following tips to find the right swimwear for your body type.

One of the best things about fashion is that it is always evolving. Now, you can mix different tops with bottoms based upon things such as color, size, prints or even fabrics. It took them a long time to understand, but swimsuit makers now see that women come in all shapes and sizes. They are built differently and need different types of swimsuit options. In addition, they like different styles, colors and patterns. When it comes to swimwear, one size does not fit all. Also, one size does not "suit" all tastes.

Be honest with yourself and look at your body. This is the only way that you'll be able to pick out the right swimsuit for yourself. Make this body assessment before you shop for your next swimsuit. Look in a full length mirror and figure out which of these body types describes you the most:

- Pear-shaped. This means that your hips flare out past your shoulders. You need swimwear that flatters your upper body and hides your bottom. Choose a solid color swimsuit. Or, try getting one that has a dark color on the bottom and a cute print on the top. At all costs, stay away from suits that have high cut legs.

- Inverted triangle. This means that you have large breasts or your shoulders are wide. You need swimwear that emphasises your bottom and ignores your top. Try to find a suit that has a square neck. This will make your shoulders look smaller. Also, prints on the bottom will draw the eye to your bottom instead of your shoulders or breasts.

- Boyish figure. This means that you have small breasts and no hips. Find swimwear that makes your body seem curvier. Swimsuits that have prints and ruffles will give you a more girlish figure. Opt for a padded halter top or a tank top and bikini bottom.

- Plus sizes. You really don't fit into any of the categories above. Find swimwear with expandable fabrics. Also, make sure that it supports your breasts and helps to hold in or camouflage your stomach.

If you are still afraid to show off your body, then purchase a swimsuit cover up. You can get a sarong, a long button down shirt, a long tee-shirt or even a wraparound skirt. These will all help to camouflage problematic body areas.

Don't forget to try on the swimsuit before purchase. Many stores will not let you return swimwear if it does not fit. It might be hard to find a swimsuit that flatters your body, but look around because it is out there.

Chapter 3: Ways to Increase Your Metabolism

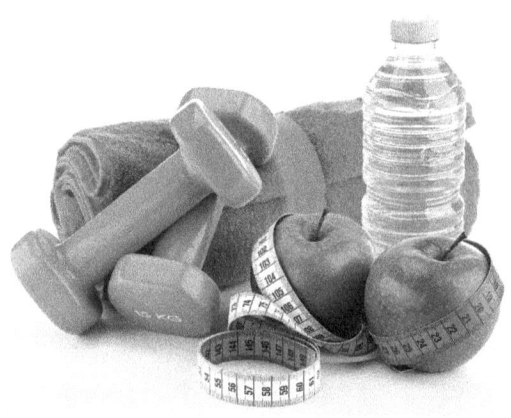

If you have been dieting and exercising, but the pounds are not melting away, there might be a problem with your metabolism. It is the main way that the body sheds the fat. You could call it a little body motor of sorts. The higher your metabolism rate, the faster you will see those pounds just drop away from your body.

As we get older, the body's metabolism rate starts to slow down. So, what needs to be done to speed up it up? Actually, there are a few things that can affect your rate in terms of weight loss. These are things such as your age and the way that you live.

Most importantly, you don't have to eat a restrictive diet just to get rid of fat. Perhaps the best way to shed those pounds and give a boost to your metabolism is to eat more food instead of eating less.

You might have to make a few changes to the way that you are doing things, but it will be worth it.

When you eat foods that are perceived to be diet foods, then you do nothing to boost your metabolism. These foods have fewer calories and are high in fiber, but you will put back on the pounds once you return to your regular way of eating.

This is because your metabolism gets out of whack whenever you diet. It no longer has the ability to kick off your metabolism like in the past. Now it is time to get it back into whack by following these simple tips:

- Eat all three of your meals. It is best to eat about four or six small meals everyday instead of skipping meals to lose weight.

- Increase your heart rate with cardio exercises. This will burn the calories and increase your metabolism as well.

- Drink eight glasses of water each day so that the water pushes out the poisons that are in your body. Toxins decrease your metabolism instead of speeding it up.

- You might think that eating carbs are bad, but they also do wonders to speed up your metabolism.

- Tone your muscles. It might help to use weights to do the trick. Try to replace excess fat with lean muscles.

- Don't eat late at night. Your body needs the day to get rid of the calories that have been consumed. If you eat at night, it does not have time to burn of those calories.

- Decrease the amount of alcohol that you drink. It also has the power to decrease your metabolism. If you must drink, do it in moderation.

Now, try all of these things to boost your metabolism. When it increases, you will be on the right road to losing weight.

Chapter 4: Fat Flushing and Increasing Your Metabolism

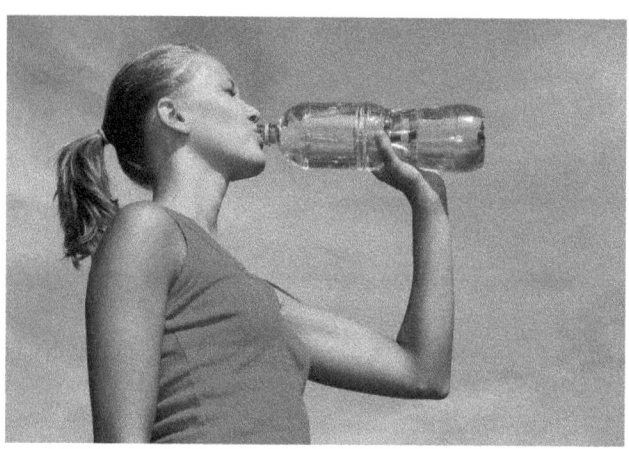

You might have to do something extreme in order to boost your metabolism. This is probably one of the few ways to burn those extra calories so that they don't turn into fat. You might also want to try flushing the fat away. This is also a good way to speed up your metabolism because it will flush toxins out of your body that tend to weigh you down and make you feel unenergetic.

Excess calories turn into fat and tend to land in three places in your body, and those places are your hips, booty and thighs. Flushing works to get the fat out of these areas. As a matter of fact, it does it much better than other diets that usually get rid of muscle too, which is definitely not a good thing.

The following are suggestions for flushing fat out of your body:

- Reduce the amount of calories that you eat. Try eating within the range of 1000 to 1500 calories per day for the first few weeks.

- Add a couple of good fats to your diet when flushing fat from your body. Try good fats such as flaxseed oil. Also eat plenty of veggies, protein and fruits. You might also want to try eating plenty of metabolism boosting spices such as cayenne pepper.

- Drink a lot of water, tea and other liquids. They do wonders to flush out the fat because they are diuretics, which get rid of toxins.

- Get plenty of rest. Sleep helps to restore the body and is needed on a nightly basis.

- Monitor your physical activity and what you eat and drink. Try writing this information in a journal, and keep it with you at all times.

Although exercise is a good thing, don't do too much of it at this time. Remember, you are consuming less food, so this will affect your energy levels for a while. Try taking a walk during your lunch time, or try hitting the treadmill after work. This should be enough physical activity.

Once the two week mark comes around, start eating 1500 calories a day. You can also add more carbs to your eating routine. Keep doing this until you have reached your goal weight. This should give your body plenty of time to increase its metabolism.

However, keep in mind that you should not decrease your caloric intake too drastically. This is not only unhealthy, but it will do nothing for permanent weight loss. Fast weight loss is hard to maintain unless you plan to eat like this for the rest of your life, which is impossible for most people to do.

The fat flushing method is ideal for anyone who has to lose a certain amount of weight by a tight deadline. For instance, you might have a class reunion, and you want to make your classmates envious. Follow this method for a few weeks, and it should help you to reach your desired weight.

CHAPTER 5: CALORIES MUST BE BURNED

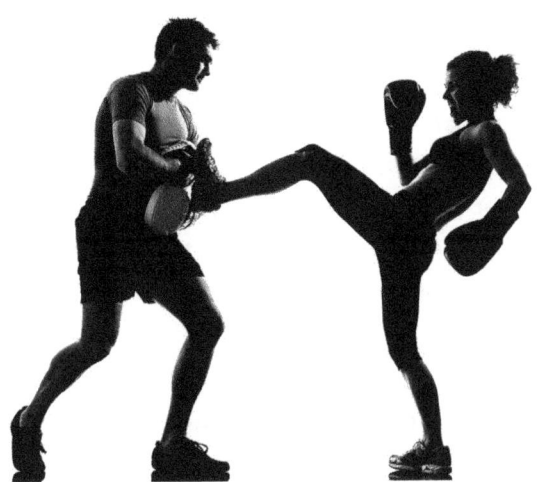

Getting off the couch and getting in shape can be achieved in a number of different ways. You can choose to join a gym, purchase exercise equipment for the home, or just commit to a regular exercise schedule that helps get you active.

Whichever way you choose to go, your ultimate goal should be to increase the amount of activities you engage in on a daily basis, as this is where you will find some real health benefits.

Invest in a Pedometer

It's not everyone who can find time in their schedule to exercise on a daily basis, but that doesn't mean you can't still lose some weight. Spending a very small amount of money on an effective little device can make all the difference.

We are talking about a pedometer and how it can help people navigate the road to weight loss. It provides an easy way to track your progress quickly and efficiently.

If you can get up to around 10,000 steps per day, you will have walked in the neighborhood of 5 miles. Eating well and using a pedometer to track your steps can help the weight come off at a steady pace. Even as you go about your regular routing, the rising number on the pedometer will show your progress.

Trying to add to that number and get it as high as possible can become habitual. You'll find that you start taking the stairs instead of the elevator, or perhaps you might park the car a block or two further away from work. As you get in better shape, you will find that these little increases become a whole lot easier to do.

Short, Sharp Bouts of Exercise at Work

Just because you are at work for 8-10 hours a day doesn't mean that you can't find ways to get some exercise. This is even true if your job requires you to sit at a desk for the duration of that time. There are still some things you can do to stay fit and healthy.

Seated leg lifts while you are seated at your desk are great. All you need to do is lift your leg, straighten it, and then count to ten before slowly lowering it back to its original position. Alternate between legs to make sure that both are properly worked.

If you have access to an office or other private space, take a few moments to do some push-ups, either on the floor standing against the wall. Sit-ups are also great if there is enough space.

When you are around the water machine or talking to another employee, take that time to so some standing leg lifts. This is done by standing one leg and bending the other at the knee. This will raise the heel of your foot to your behind, which is a pose that you be held for a ten count. Alternate this exercise between legs.

Use your lunch break to go for a nice brisk walk around the office. If the weather is nice, head outside and walk around the block. Another great way to get your walk in and your step count up is to walk to the office where you need to deliver a message as opposed to typing out an email.

As mentioned earlier, take the stairs instead of the elevator, as this is a great workout. Switch out the chair at your desk with an exercise ball. Your abdominal and calf muscles with both get a workout when going this route. It may seem uncomfortable at first, so use the ball for short periods to start with and build up your time each day.

Toe raises are another simple exercise you can do at your desk. Leave your heel planted firmly on the ground and lift your toes for a count of ten. Lower and start again with the other foot.

You can shape your behind and burn calories by squeezing your glutes. This can be done any time you are standing around, or you can even do it while you are in the restroom.

There are a number of other exercises that you can easily perform at the office, with jumping jacks, lunges, and running in place just a few that will help you burn calories. Take a few minutes for each during the day will quickly add up to a full workout.

Turn Cleaning Into an Exercise Routine

Life can often get in the way of making it to the gym, but that doesn't mean that you have to give up on exercising altogether. If you have spent some time building up an exercise routine, skipping a few days can make you end up quitting completely.

On those days that you can't make it to the gym, you need to find way to get a workout in. Cleaning is a great way to do that, as you will be moving and burning calories. If you feel the urge to skip the gym, decide to clean the house instead.

Cleaning is just like working out in that the more vigorous the activity, the more calories you can burn. Sweeping the floor in a single room can burn as many as 112 calories. Moving on to vacuuming can lead to another 119 calories being burned.

Getting the duster out and general tidying can burn 85 calories. Another 68 calories can be used up in making your bed. All of the cleaning tasks we have mentioned so far, which doesn't add up to a whole lot of work, can burn a very nice 272 calories.

If that work took about an hour, there is a good chance your calories burned would be doubled. Just doing laundry will burn about 36 calories for every 15 minutes of activity.

Scrubbing the floors can really burn up some calories. On average, you can expect to burn 258 calories for every hour that you spend scrubbing.

Spring cleaning will burn a ton of calories and will give you a great workout that would be akin to spending time on a treadmill at pretty high speeds. Even the easier cleaning chores will burn calories. For example, washing the dishes by hand will use up 78 calories.

Cleaning that makes you sweat is where the calories can really be used up. Giving the bathroom a thorough cleaning will burn 200 calories for every half hour of activity. If you live in a larger home that has more than one bathroom, you can multiply that calorie count by the number of bathrooms to get the total amount burned.

One of the biggest advantages about burning calories while you clean, besides having a sparkling home, is that the tasks can be broken up over the course of a day as opposed to doing it all at once.

It's a good idea to commit to cleaning for 10-15 minute burst throughout the day. You don't have to do it for hours at a time to reap the benefits.

Taking Your Calorie Burning Activities Outdoors

If you run out of things to do inside your home, you can always go outside to burn calories. One great way to do that is to take your dog for a walk, which is an activity that can very easily result in you burning as much as 150 calories every half hour.

There are plenty of things to do on the outside that will help make your house look nice and burn calories in the process. Getting the water out and washing your windows will see you burn off about 102 calories every half hour.

One of the quickest ways to burn calories with outside activities is mowing the lawn. If you tip the scales at 200 pounds or more, you can easily burn 276 calories per half hour when you mow the lawn. Just imagine how many you could burn if you live on a large piece of land.

Make the car look like new again can help you burn about 204 calories per hour. Gardening is more than just mowing the lawn, which is good news for those that love to plant flowers. Adding a little floral color can result in 272 calories burned off every hour.

Get Healthy While Having Fun

Burning calories can often feel like hard work, but that doesn't have to be the case. There are plenty of fun activities that you can engage in that will help you burn calories. Sign up for a dancing class, or simply get the music on and dance around your home.

No matter where you choose to dance, you can bet that the calories will come off. You can easily burn off 240 calories per half hour by dancing, depending of course on what style of dance you engage in. Complex, faster paced dancing will see you burn calories on the high end of the scale.

If you have a roller skating rink in your area, you can burn off 350 calories per half hour while you have some real fun. If you like a sportier way to burn calories, think about taking a kickboxing class. You can burn off 480 calories every half hour performing that activity.

That adds up to almost 1,000 calories if you engage in an hour long class. It's a fantastic way to get in shape, plus you also learn some effective self-defense techniques.

Racquet sports like tennis, squash, and badminton are excellent in helping you burn calories quickly. Squash is the fastest paced of the three, and thus allows you to burn more calories. You can expect to burn 533 calories for every half hour you play.

Tennis is the next best with 400 calories every half hour, followed by badminton at 285 calories. Bowling is another way to burn calories, at a rate of about 308 per hour. Golf is slower paced, but if you walk the course, you will cover about five miles on average.

There will still be days when the thought of doing anything just isn't that appealing. On those days, take some time to play with your kids or pets, as that fun activity will allow you to burn off about 241 calories or more.

CHAPTER 6: GET TO KNOW THE BASICS OF WEIGHT LOSS

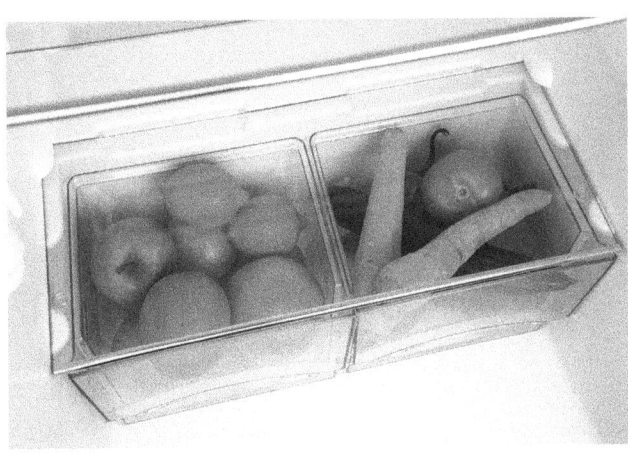

Before you can effectively lose weight, a basic idea of how calories work is required. Calories are the energy your body gets when you eat, which it then uses like fuel. If you use a fireplace analogy, adding too much wood to the fire can mean that heat is produced in excess.

The same rules apply with food. If you eat too much, you will end up with large reserves of unused fuel. All that wood you have chopped and stacked by the fire is similar to how your body stacks and stores excess calories, which in turns into fat for easier storage.

Your body needs places to put that fat, so it tends to go to spots you'd rather it would not. That's when you end up with a double chin or excess weight hanging over the waist band of your pants. As if the appearance of the fat weren't b ad enough, it can look even worse when cellulite gives it a lumpy, cottage cheese like look.

Cellulite is actually pockets of fat that sit right below the surface of the skin. It's an accumulation of all those foods you shouldn't eat that end up as unburned calories.

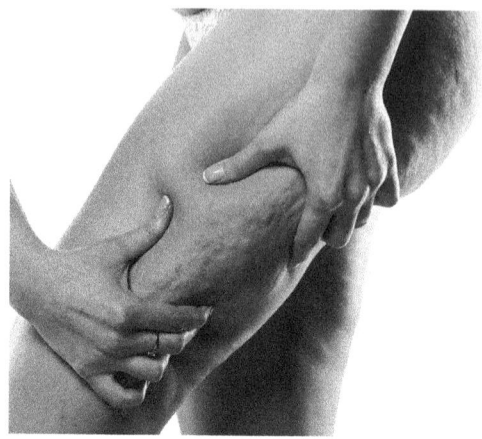

If truth be told, most people give little thought to the consequences when they sit down to have a meal. We are all aware of the foods that are not good for us and what will happen if we eat too much of them. Ingesting too much unhealthy food leads to weight gain.

Every time you put food in your mouth, your body sets about the task of digesting it. A bunch of energy is burned when your body does this, giving it an invisible workout. On the face of things, a workout without the work sounds like a dream come true.

Just think about it: you are hanging out on the couch watching television or chilling in some other way, and your body is burning energy. Isn't that just perfect?

If its' so great, then why are so many people still carrying excess weight? It all comes down to the foods that you choose to eat. Portion measuring, carb counting, and labeling foods as good or bad is standard practice.

The reality is that good and bad doesn't apply, as all food is nothing but fuel. How quickly the fuel is used up depends on the foods you eat and how your body responds to it.

Negative Calorie Foods - Your Body's Best Friend

Imagine being able to lose weight by simply eating the right types of foods. You might think of foods that burn calories just by eating them as some sort of magic, but they do exist. There are in fact foods that make your body use more energy to digest them than the calories they contain.

Foods that take more energy to digest than the calories they contain are referred to as negative calorie foods. Eating these foods regularly will mean that you will burn calories and lose weight.

Let's take a look at how it all plays out:

You feel like having a sweet snack when you are out and about and end up settling for a 350 calorie slice of cake. The moment that the last piece of that delicious cake crosses your lips, your body sets about the process of digesting it.

If we are being generous, let's say that your body burns off 150 calories during that burning process. That still leaves an excess of 200 calories resting in your bodies. If they remain unused, they will be stored as fat and cause weight gain. Keep in mind, the amount of calories burned with negative calorie foods will depend entirely on what type of food you eat.

Let's imagine that there is an apple for sale beside that slice of cake. If you choose the apple, you are looking at about 80 calories, with the digestion process beginning when you eat it.

Your body has a harder digestion job ahead of it due to the fact that apples are negative calories foods. If you compare what it takes to digest the apple and the cake, you are looking at the difference between walking and running. A nice stroll around your neighborhood is not going to burn as much energy as it would if you had ran the same distance.

Breaking Down the Numbers

There aren't a lot of people who love to do math, but we can assure you, these are numbers you will like. Again, that apple you ate means an ingestion of 80 calories or so. Your body begins the silent workout process of digesting it.

On average, it takes about 105 calories, give or take a few, to digest that 80 calorie apple. The math then tells you that it took an extra 25 calories just to digest that single apple.

If you had gone with the slice of cake, but also added an apple into the mix, you would have essentially saved 25 calories on the cake portion. That would then mean that the 350 calorie slice of cake, which would usually leave the excess of 200 calories, would now be down to an excess of 175. You are still taking in more calories than you burn in digesting, but the scales are tipping more in your favor when you add negative calorie foods.

The math is not quite that basic when you have been eating the wrong way for months or even years. By regularly adding negative calorie foods into your diet, you can start to lose weight and undo some of the damage done over the years.

As is the case with any type of diet, there is a little more involved in the process. If you adopt a diet that is complicated or difficult to follow, the chances are better than average that you won't see it through. Simple and easy is the best way to weight loss success.

You may have heard about food journals where you record everything you eat, as well as the amount of calories in each thing. It's a good idea in principal, but keeping it up over a long period is difficult. Negative calorie foods are a simple way to get the weight loss process off and running, as well as being easy to maintain for a long time.

Your body wants to help, and it can do that by you putting the right types of foods into your digestive system. This will allow you to out the numbers in your favor.

Breaking into the Store

If you are someone that loves to eat, you may well have more than your fair share of excess fat being stored. It's all about the numbers again, as you need to start eating negative calorie foods if you want to get rid of that fat. Simply put, those foods will act like thieves going into your store and stealing the supplies.

Once they get their hands on that fat, they are going to start putting it to use. This happens because you are using up more energy to digest the food than it brought to the table. The difference has to be made up, which means the stored fat is taken in order to do that.

When negative calorie foods are ingested, your body essentially negates the calories when it goes to work pulling out the nutrients and energy it needs. If your body can't find enough energy in the food to complete the process, it will head to the fat stores and start to fill its basket. It won't stop until the energy required has been used up.

Are These Negative Calorie Foods Healthy?

There is usually always a catch with something this good, right? The negative calorie foods we are talking about probably taste awful or are really hard to find. Worse yet, they probably just aren't that good for you, right?

Wrong!

Not only are negative calorie foods healthy, doctors and dieticians recommend that you get as many of these foods into your diet as possible if you want to maintain your weight and stay healthy. So, what exactly are these magic foods? They are, for the most part, fruits and vegetables, which are an essential part of any weight loss plan.

To list all of the foods that fall into the negative calorie category would take more space than we have here, but let's take a look at just a few on the vegetable list: turnips, cucumbers, lettuce, asparagus, broccoli, radishes, cabbage, celery, spinach, carrots, leeks and cauliflower.

If you aren't big on veggies, there are plenty of fruits to choose from, including: watermelon, apricot, tomato, apple, blackberry, tangerine, cranberry, cantaloupe, peaches, lime, grapefruit, lemon, papaya, honeydew melon, strawberries, pineapple, plums, mandarin orange, raspberry, rhubarb and honeydew melon.

As you can see, these are all foods that are readily available at your local grocery store. They are affordable, delicious foods that are good for you. One mistake that you should not make is thinking that there are no calories in these foods, as that is not the case.

There are indeed calories in these foods, but the energy that your body has to generate to digest them is where you essentially negate those calories completely.

Are these types of foods safe to consume?

Absolutely!! When was the last time you heard about someone overdosing on a fruit plate? Unlike many of the "miracle weight loss" products on the market, there is nothing found in these foods that can do you any harm. Losing weight and staying healthy can be achieved by adding negative calorie foods into your diet.

Chapter 7: Supplements – Are They Right for You?

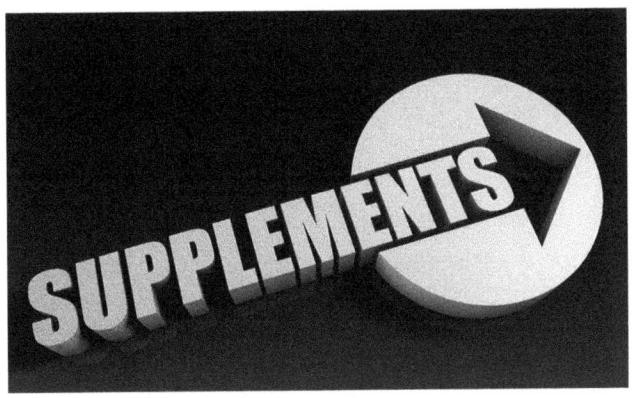

Try to find a nutritious program that you can follow with ease. Also, try to find an exercise plan that works for you. Take it even further and use supplements that can help you to reach your goal.

Supplements: Be Cautious

If you plan to use supplements, be conscious of the foods and drinks that you consume. You don't want dangerous food and drink combinations that could make you unhealthy. Research various supplements and be forewarned that you are going to hear a lot of debateable information about them.

The use of supplements is debated among professionals within the dietary industry. Some think that supplements are okay. For instance, Dr. Oz is always promoting the benefits of using green coffee bean extract, but other professionals would probably argue that it is not safe to use.

However, most experts in the dietary industry would prefer that your nutrition is obtain from real foods and beverages, and not supplements. It is not wise to just consume sodas, pills and fast foods on a regular basis. Obviously, it is not healthy to eat like this.

Good Results versus Taking Good Care of Yourself

Keep in mind that you should also take good care of yourself, which can be done on a budget. Not all splurges have to be expensive. You don't always have to have fancy massages in order to take good care of yourself.

Simple things such as reading a good book, or scheduling a time and place for a little rest and relaxation can help you to feel wonderful.

Find motivation via your favorite blogs and books. They can help you to get inspired and to ignore negative and depressing information.

Chapter 8: Fighting a Flabby Tummy in Search of 6 Pack Abs

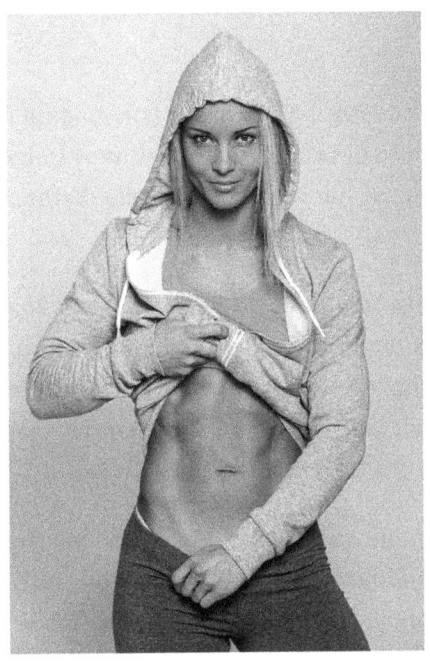

Are you one of those people who have a decent looking body save for that little roll of flab around the middle that likes to stubbornly stick around? You may give it a cute name like your spare tire, but the reality is that it's fat that is getting in the way of the 6 pack abs that are hiding underneath just waiting to be set free.

The first step in getting rid of that fat is to reduce the amount of calories that you take in on a daily basis. Furthermore, the calories you do get should include foods that have proven to be fat burners. Those include such items as veggies and lean protein. Carbohydrates should be reduced, especially in the evening when your metabolism is shutting down for the night. Go for low-fat options as often as possible and let those abs get out where they belong.

What's important to understand is that ab toning and fat loss is not the same thing. You can tone your abs with the right exercise, but in order to lose that excess fat, you need to attack from the inside out. Spot reduction exercises will do nothing to burn the fat around your waist.

The weight loss industry will try to sell you magical pills and potions that are designed to get rid of a flabby tummy quickly, but they are a waste of money, as hard work is the only currency your belly will accept.

That doesn't mean you need to ignore the abs that lay below the fat. As you work on your diet, you should also be doing exercises meant to work the abs. It is important to choose the right exercise for the job, and you may be surprised to learn that tummy crunches are not the best choice you can make.

Before you commit to an exercise schedule, figure out which exercises work and how to do them properly. Just as important as the proper technique is how you breathe while you work out. Search online and you will find a ton of great information about great abdominal exercises.

Resistance training is an excellent way to work on your abs. If you have back issues, make sure to use an exercise ball for support when you work out. There is no reason to go overboard either, so limit your exercise schedule to about three days per week to begin with.

A good cardio workout is also a great way to burn fat, so be sure to mix some cardio exercise into the mix once you get started. Cardio exercises are best done in the morning before you eat, making sure to work both the upper and lower body when you do.

Keep in mind that real results take time, so don't get discouraged if your progress is slow. You just have to keep working and digging under the fat to get to those 6 pack abs.

Work On Your Arms When You Exercise

If you avoid wearing sleeveless dresses or tops because you are self-conscious about flabby arms, you are not alone. This is actually a common problem for those who lose weight, as the skin sticks around long after the fat cells are gone.

The arms are actually one of the most difficult parts of the body to firm and tone, which is why it's better to just exercise the whole body as opposed to targeting flabby arms. Fat cells love to gather in the arms more than anywhere else, so use aerobic exercise to lose fat and tone the arms at the same time.

Working on the biceps and triceps is required if you want firm, sexy arms. The front of your arm is where the biceps are stored, while the triceps make their home around back. When you build up both of those muscles, you will be adding depth that will fill up that saggy skin.

Exercise bands and weights are all you need to get on the road to those sexy arms. The following three exercises should definitely be included in your exercise routine:

Exercise #1 – Place the middle of the exercise band under your feet and grasp the ends of the band in both hands. Bend one elbow from the waist, with the band stretching up and forward. Your biceps will start to tense when the band is raised. Repeat the movement about 8 to 10 times on each arm, keeping your elbow slightly bent each time.

Exercise #2 – Repeat the exercise listed above, only this time pull the band out from the left and right side of your body 8 to 10 times for each arm.

Exercise #3 – Repeat the same process as above, only this time the band gets pulled backwards on either side of your body. The triceps will get a real workout with this one.

Weights are another great way to get your arms in shape. No need to pump iron here, as you can start out with smaller weights that you use while sitting or lying on the floor.

The most effective arm exercises are those that provide resistance to the triceps and biceps, as that helps with toning. Pilates has also proven to be effective in shaping the arms, so look for yoga or Pilate's websites that have a list of arm exercises.

You won't have to work overly hard to see positive results, and the good news is that you tend to see them pretty quickly, too.

Turn to Exercise to Prevent Sagging Breasts

The vast majority of women, especially those of the larger breasted variety, are likely to experience the discomfort of seeing their breasts start to sag. Age is usually the culprit here, but the reality is that there is no time frame for the sagging to begin.

There are no muscles to be found in the breasts, but rather a large network of connective tissue and ligaments. The job of these parts is to effectively deliver milk to newborns, with the result of that being that the tissues shrivel and cause the breasts to sag. Women without children will not escape the sagging, though, as they will still lose the elasticity in the skin that helps keep the breasts upright and perky.

What's even more disconcerting is that bras do little to prevent the sagging. There has in fact been research done that shows that wearing a bra may actually speed up the sagging process. This is because they remain immobile when housed in a bra, causing an atrophy of sorts. What the bra does will is lift and shapes the breasts to make them more attractive under your clothing.

It is possible to keep the breasts toned and sagging at bay using the following exercises:

* **Push-ups** – This is a great exercise for your entire upper body, not just your breasts. If pushing up from floor level is too much, try doing them against a wall.

* **Chest presses** – Weights or stretch bands can be employed to work on the pectoral muscles, which will leave your breasts looking form and fabulous.

The fact of the matter is that all good upper body exercises will have a positive effect on your breasts. If you decide to start jogging, invest in a quality sports bra. The constant bouncing caused by jogging could damage the ligaments and actually speed up the sagging process.

If you want to feel good about your breasts and your body, stand up straight in front of a mirror. You will notice that your breasts raise up naturally, which shows the importance of good posture.

Keeping the skin healthy also helps, so get in the habit of exfoliating and applying lotion to your breasts. Good nutrition is also a must, as a healthy diet will help keep the ligaments healthy as you get older, which will help prevent sagging.

Maintaining a healthy weight also helps keep your breasts looking their best. Excess weight tends to put gravity into action, with the breasts being just one of the victims. Yes, your bra size may drop, but your breasts will stay up and perky through it all.

Move Your Way To A Firmer Butt!

You can bet that most women have, at one point or another in their life, asked if their butt looks big in a particular outfit. Of all the female body parts, the butt may be the one that women give the most thought to. It seems as though the search is constantly on for that one garment that will make the butt look absolutely perfect, which in turn leads to a spike in self-confidence.

Like it or not, the backside is home to a very large number of fat cells, and it's a place where they are all quite happy to live. If you want a butt that is tight and looks great in any garment, you are not going to get there without a good deal of hard work.

None of the great butt-shaping exercise routines that are out there will make a lick of difference if you don't also incorporate a fat burning diet program. You will also need a healthy dose of desire and determination if your butt is to look its very best.

You don't have to shell out on expensive exercise equipment or a gym membership to get your butt in shape. Waking and/or jogging can help with toning, as well as being a great cardio option. Riding a bike or playing active sports like tennis, volleyball, or swimming can also help.

The two very best butt shaping exercises are as follows:

Front Lunges – Placing your feet shoulder length apart, take a step forward with your left foot. You should bend at the knee and move your leg forward until the knee is directly over the ankle. Move back to your stating position before repeating the move with your right leg. Use a chair for support if needed.

Squats – Move your feet apart, keep your back straight, and get into a squat position. Move slowly back to your original position and then repeat. Your first few attempts may require the use of a chair for balance. You can squat until your butt hits the chair before going back to the original position.

Kickboxing is a great way to mix things up if you get tired of your regular toning exercises. If you have a gym membership, you'll likely notice that they now offer kickboxing classes. The movements used in the kicks are a great aerobic exercise, as well as the perfect way to firm the butt.

You will never have to ask the big butt question again of you commit some time and effort into exercises that tone and shape your behind.

Adding Definition to Your Leg Muscles

There are those who have naturally great looking legs, whereas the rest of us have to work to get the definition we desire. The good news is that there are plenty of great exercises that can help make it happen. The most effective exercises tend to be those that combine strength training with fat-burning cardio routines that target the legs.

A good leg program usually incorporates cardio exercise a few times per week. Squats, lunges, and calf raises are the exercises most commonly used to define the leg muscles.

Sports that require the use of the legs are the best at helping you get the strength and muscle definition that you want. Tennis, skiing, and swimming are just a few of the sports that will add curves to your legs and help you look great in shorts and skirts.

An effective leg workout can be achieved with a treadmill or a step back to nature with a brisk outdoor walk. An exercise mat or workout bench can come in handy, as can an exercise ball. All of these will allow you to stretch your leg muscles to the max.

Some of the most effective toning exercise for the legs are:

- Squats – Bend the knees and keep your back straight for a count of 10. Perform 5 reps.

- Kicks – Lie stomach down on your exercise ball and kick upwards, 3 times for each leg.

- Outer thigh lifts – Using a chair for balance, lift each leg outward 5 times.

Exercise will help you achieve great looking legs, but if you are carrying excess weight, you will also need to try and reduce your body fat in order to get the best results. A fat-burning diet in combination with your exercise schedule will produce the very best results.

The best diet that you can adopt is one that is balanced, as this will burn fat and boost your metabolism. A good daily helping of fruits and vegetables is a must. With your fruit selections, chose those that are high in Vitamin C, such as grapefruits, limes, lemons, and oranges.

Other helpful fruits include apples and berries, which the body has to use more energy to digest. These fruits also contain something called pectin, which essentially limits the amount of fat cells that can be absorbed by your body. It's also important to drink plenty of water to flush out toxins and prevent cramping when you exercise.

With a little hard work and determination, your legs will be looking great in shorts and skirts before you know it.

CHAPTER 9: TIPS ON MOTIVATION AND STAYING ON TRACK

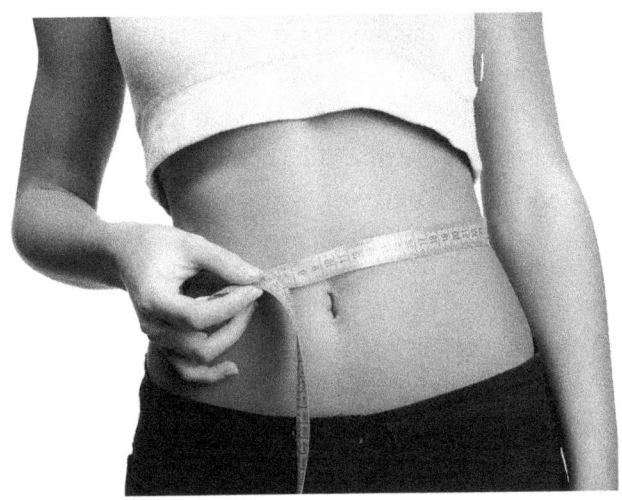

Many times you might feel hopeless when it comes to your new fitness program. But there are ways to monitor your fitness goals and keep you on track so that you'll remain motivated and get good results.

Try weighing yourself just once a month instead of doing it weekly or daily. This will give you something to look forward to and also allow you to see the payoff for everything that you have done for the month. You won't be as depressed when you don't see weekly progress.

You might also want to monitor your weight loss by taking your body measurements. Many times the scale is not a good indicator of what is really going on with your body. A scale cannot show the inches that have been lost due to your hard work. Taking your measurements will allow you to see that your hard work is really paying off.

Take your measurements when you are naked. If you want to know how to take your measurements, then find a few measurement charts that can help. Get into the habit of measuring yourself a minimum of once a week or once a month.

You can also monitor the amount of body fat that your body has. This will tell you how much fat you need to get rid of in order to reach your desired goal weight. For women the percentage of body fat should be in the range of 25 to 31 percent. For men it should be in the range of 18 to 25 percent.

You can measure the amount of fat that your body has by using hydrostatic weighing, DEXA, callipers and bioelectrical impedance scales. However, the easiest way to measure your body fat is by using an online calculator that utilizes a tap measurement or the skin fold. If you are a health club member, inquire about the health club's methods for measuring body fat.

One of the best ways to get motivated is to actually see yourself at your desired goal weight. This can be done via a digitally enhanced before and after picture of yourself. You might have to dish out some money to have this done, but it will be well worth it. This is especially true if it works to keep you motivated. This is a great way to make you stick to your diet plan and exercise.

Look online and find a site that produces digitally enhanced photos. All you have to do is upload a photo of yourself, the company then digitally reduces your size on the photo. You will receive your new digitally enhanced photo via email.

Take this photo and put it on your refrigerator door or a bedroom mirror for motivation. Now you can really see what you will look like if you lose that unwanted body fat, which should motivate you even more.

MEET THE AUTHOR

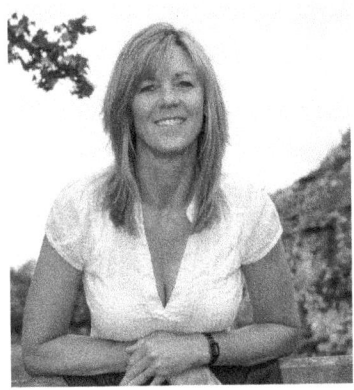

Zoey Taylor leads her clients towards better health and fitness, not unrealistic bodies, diets and workout routines. Sometimes that means lifestyle changes, hardcore training, and motivational triggers and sometimes it means addressing medical complexities through nutrition and stress management. Zoey has years of experience in the areas of health, fitness and nutrition. She uses her experience in these areas to help people with diet, fitness and improving their overall health and happiness.

Zoey struggled with weight and body image issues as a teenager. In college she began to study nutrition and implemented what she was learning in her own diet. Through diet and fitness Zoey shed her larger self and has never looked back. Zoey's weight struggles gave her an appreciation for what overweight people struggle with on a daily basis. After college Zoey took her knowledge to the next level by becoming a certified personal trainer and nutritionist.

Zoey resides in Sunny California and is an outdoor enthusiast. Zoey loves to stay fit - hiking, snowboarding, swimming and has become an avid tennis player. Zoey and her husband Art enjoy traveling to new places, campfires on the beach and good wine.

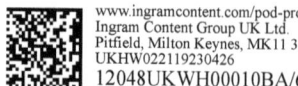
www.ingramcontent.com/pod-product-compliance
Ingram Content Group UK Ltd.
Pitfield, Milton Keynes, MK11 3LW, UK
UKHW022119230426
12048UKWH00010BA/612